Breaking the Sugar Habit:
Practical Ways to Cut the Sugar, Lose the Weight, and Regain Your Health

MARGARET WERTHEIM, MS, RD

The information contained in this book is for informational purposes only and is not intended to replace professional medical advice. Consult with your doctor before making any changes to your diet. If you have a medical problem, you should seek medical care from a qualified healthcare provider.

Mention of specific organizations, associations or experts does not indicate an endorsement, nor should mention of these entities be interpreted as endorsement of this book.

Cover design by Elizabeth Haight.

Find FREE recipes and tips at Sugarbreaker.com/resources

ISBN-13: 978-1495380907
ISBN-10: 1495380904

For my Dad who knew sugar was the problem all along.

PREFACE

I wrote this book for all the patients, clients, and friends I see struggling with health problems caused by sugar on a daily basis. Most people have been trained to fixate on reducing fat and are less conscious of their sugar intake. Others try to reduce their sugar intake, but struggle with cravings or are unsure how little or how much sugar is acceptable to have. I'd like to address both of these problems. I start with the former, establishing the link between high intakes of sugar in the diet and weight gain and diseases like diabetes, heart disease, metabolic syndrome, and cancer. Heart disease and cancer are two diseases most people would associate with excessive fat intake, but there is mounting evidence that sugar plays a role in their development. I suspect if I were to stop people on the street and ask them what causes diabetes, most people would resoundingly say "sugar." The prevailing idea in the medical community is that diabetes is actually caused by being overweight or obese (combined with some genetic factors). In many cases, becoming overweight or obese happened as a result of excess sugar intake. The high sugar intake led to weight gain and the two together contributed to the development of diabetes.

For many years, the target of public health campaigns has been fat, and that eating fat must cause you to accumulate fat on your body – a logical conclusion if only our bodies operated so simply. Especially since fat is higher in calories than sugar with 9 calories per gram compared to the 4 calories per gram of protein or carbohydrate, it would make sense that eating fat makes you fat. Unfortunately, this line of thinking is much too simplistic. It ignores the fact that excess sugar is converted to fat by the body in a process triggered by the hormone insulin. The higher your carbohydrate and sugar intake, the higher your insulin levels, the more fat is stored by your body. When weight loss is the goal, cutting sugar intake should always be the first step in order to lower insulin levels. The fact that fat is high in calories *does* matter, but it isn't the only thing that matters. I will show you the research on the negative health impacts of sugar, fructose, and artificial sweeteners. Then we'll move toward practical solutions for reducing sugar in your diet and healthier alternative sweeteners to use. Lastly I'll provide some dessert and beverage recipes to try that are low in added sugar and naturally nutrient-rich. At the end of each of the four parts of this book, you will find a summary of key points for that section and actionable items.

You should know that I don't intend to say that you should never eat a piece of cake again at a birthday party or eat some apple crisp at a dinner party. These are enjoyable parts of life that should be savored *on occasion, but not every day*. For most people, the problem with sweets is that they eat them every day after lunch and dinner or just generally too frequently. Even if you aren't drinking soda or eating lots of desserts, you may be eating non-dessert foods with added sugar like instant oatmeal, crackers, protein and granola bars, and yogurt, all of which may be detrimental. My goal is not to take away pleasure, but to strike the right balance so that your daily practices promote health and well-being instead of disease and loss of quality of life. I have seen things I wish I hadn't seen and wish didn't exist in the world – loss of mobility due to obesity, loss of limbs to amputation from uncontrolled diabetes, kidney failure necessitating a lifetime of dialysis, and infertility associated with obesity.

On an encouraging note, I have seen a client lose 80 pounds in a year after giving up a daily soda habit and drastically cutting sugar and refined carbs. Results like this are possible, but you'll have to find ways to choose long-term success and health over the short-term pleasure of a soda or a piece of cake. Instead you'll have to find short-term pleasure in having steady energy levels and mood, or watching the pounds fall off. Disease prevention is not always a very good motivator when you are healthy. It often takes a health problem to spur people to action, but I hope you'll look around you and be motivated by the preventable conditions of others. Not every health problem is preventable, but so many are. If you are thin and healthy now, I hope the desire for longevity and vibrant health will spur you to action. I also want to emphasize that I don't intend to ignore or downplay the detrimental role of other refined carbohydrates and excess overall carbohydrates. These can be very problematic too, but that is beyond the scope of this book and limiting sugar should always be the first step towards better health.

This book is for anyone who struggles with sugar cravings, realizes the problem, and wants to decrease their sugar intake once and for all. On the other hand, perhaps you are overweight and have tried low-fat diets without success. Then this book is for you. The final group I'm speaking to is healthcare providers and health coaches. Getting your patients and clients to cut their sugar intake is one of the most valuable things you can do for their health. I designed this book to provide you with well-researched information so that you can start to have those conversations with your patients and clients on why sugar is harmful and why it's important to limit. For the physicians out there: you have tremendous power with your patients. If you tell them that sugar is a major cause of their health problems, they will listen. Communicating the link to your patients, and then referring them to a registered dietitian nutritionist or qualified health coach who can really help them change, is a powerful step.

TABLE OF CONTENTS

INTRODUCTION

The World Health Organization defines health as follows – "health is a state of complete physical, mental and social well-being and not merely the absence of disease or infirmity (1)." This book is designed to help you achieve that higher level of physical well-being through improving your diet. One of the most wonderful things about being a nutritionist is seeing that one positive change tends to lead to another. Improvements in physical well-being tend to lead to improvements in mental and social well-being as well.

We're focusing on sugar, and I want to show you what a big problem sugar consumption is in the US. According to the United States Department of Agriculture (USDA), the average American consumed 76 pounds of sugar in 2012 with 39 pounds being refined cane or beet sugar, 27 pounds from high fructose corn syrup, and 10 pounds from other sweeteners (2). This is equivalent to 94 grams of added sugar every day, well above even the most lax agency's recommendations on sugar consumption. Believe it or not, this is actually a decline in sugar consumption in the US! The majority of this sugar comes from soda, energy drinks, and sports drinks followed by grain-based desserts like cakes, cookies, and pies (3). Ninety-four grams of sugar provide 375 calories every day - nutrient-lacking, health-destroying calories causing weight gain, diabetes, and tooth decay.

According to a 2011 Gallup poll, about 30% of Americans are trying to lose weight at any given time (4). If you are one of those people and you eat sugar and drink sugar-sweetened beverages daily, drastically cutting your sugar intake is a very effective way to lose weight, more so than the popular low-fat diets. Even if you are thin, whether you feel awful or well, are active or inactive, you can still be setting yourself up for health problems down the road with a high intake of sugar. This book is not targeted only to people who are trying to lose weight. There are skinny diabetics, and there are people who are thin with heart disease, cancer and other health problems. In an age when so many people are overweight, it's important to realize that thin does not mean healthy. As you will read throughout this book, sugar has direct detrimental health effects independent of its ability to cause weight gain, overweight, and obesity.

Attitudes toward sugar are changing, albeit slowly. The rise of Paleolithic and lower carbohydrate diets and the failure of low-fat and high carb diets as effective weight loss strategies have helped. People are starting to see that sugar and refined carbohydrates are problematic for their health. If I were to ask a person on the street what causes heart disease, the answer would probably be bacon, french fries, or lard. I can't imagine someone saying "coke" or "sugar." But the reality is that sugar and refined carbohydrates are part of the heart disease process through the development of metabolic syndrome, which I will discuss later. It's apparent attitudes are changing. Mark Bittman, author of *How to Cook Everything* and *Food Matters* writes in his opinion piece in the *New York Times* entitled, "It's the Sugar, Folks," that in fact, according to a new study sugar may cause diabetes independently of weight (5). Marion Nestle, on her *Food Politics* blog, doesn't go so far as to say sugar causes diabetes, but she does note, "Although a small percentage of overweight people develop type 2 diabetes, most people with type 2 diabetes are overweight. Losing weight is the first thing to do to prevent or treat type 2 diabetes. Reducing intake of sugary sodas is the first thing to do to lose weight (6)." Most members of the healthcare and medical community still won't say sugar causes diabetes, out of respect to evidence-based medicine. In evidence-based medicine, the research needs to show clear evidence of benefit or risk from a certain behavior or drug, or screening method, before it is incorporated into routine practice. While I consider myself committed to providing nutrition information that is based on science and not merely conjecture, I feel comfortable saying that there is a very good chance that sugar increases risk of diabetes and other chronic diseases. When there is no good coming from sugar (aside from temporary pleasure) and likely harm, I think the necessary action is clear!

That's not to say that physicians and dietitians ever thought sugar was healthy or good for you, but I just don't think the harm that sugar causes has been demonstrated clearly enough. I remember the weight loss advice that claimed it better to eat some jellybeans instead of ice cream, since the jellybeans are lower in calories. I'm sure there are still some people out there giving this terrible advice. Yes, jellybeans are lower in calories, but they have absolutely no vitamins or minerals and are loaded with sugar and artificial colors. As I will show you later, jellybeans have a high glycemic index, spiking blood sugar and insulin levels, which can lead to fat storage and potentially diabetes development. In the meantime, ice cream has a very low glycemic index and actually has some nutritional value with calcium, potassium and vitamin A. I'm not promoting ice cream as a health food or saying you should eat it frequently. I think the important point is that optimum health is not achieved by meeting an exact calorie goal, but instead is attained by eating whole, real and unrefined foods in proper proportions.

If you are accustomed to eating sugar every day, the process of weaning yourself off of it will not be painless, and may be slow, unless you have the determination to quit cold turkey. It's a worthy cause, because it can help you regain and improve your health and well-being. Without good health, enjoyment of life and following your dreams is that much harder. We all have varying degrees of health potential. Some people are struck with diseases that seem to have no rhyme or reason, but many diseases are preventable with the proper diet and lifestyle measures. One of the best things you can do for your health is to quit sugar in order to have more energy, reduce your risk of chronic disease, and live longer and more vibrantly.

Part 1: Everything You Don't Know About Sugar

CHAPTER 1: SUGAR BASICS

Let me start out by answering the question, "what is sugar?" This question does not have a simple straightforward answer. Sugar comes in different forms, each of which behaves differently in the body. Sugars are the building blocks of carbohydrates. They are made up of carbon, hydrogen, and oxygen atoms. Your body breaks down sugar into carbon dioxide and water in order to provide energy for your body.

The word "sugar" refers to several different compounds. The simple sugars, called monosaccharides, consist of a single molecular unit. Glucose and fructose are monosaccharides. Disaccharides are composed of two monosaccharide units linked together. Sucrose, the disaccharide found in table sugar, is a combination of glucose and fructose. Other less common disaccharides are lactose, made up of glucose and galactose, and maltose, which is composed of two glucose molecules. Glucose, fructose, and sucrose are found in varying amounts in fruits, some starchy vegetables like carrots, desserts, and sweeteners (7).

Added sugars in foods include those from refined white sugar, rapadura, evaporated cane juice, brown sugar, powdered sugar, whole cane sugar, honey, molasses, maple syrup, agave nectar, brown rice syrup, coconut sugar, date sugar, beet sugar, and high fructose corn syrup. Of course some sweeteners are better than others due to their differing combinations of sugar molecules, different impact on blood sugar levels, and variances in vitamin, mineral, and antioxidant content. In the end, these are all sources of sugar that have negative health consequences when consumed in excess. In Chapter 11, I discuss the best sweeteners to use, but the main objective is to use only small amounts of any type of sweetener, because sugar, no matter what the form, has health consequences, as you will learn in Chapter 5.

Complex carbohydrates (carbs for short) are made up of many glucose molecules linked together. Examples of complex carbs are those that make up grains, legumes, vegetables, and potatoes. These complex carbs are broken down during the process of digestion into 100% glucose. This is markedly different from foods that contain added or natural sugars, as these foods contain a combination of glucose, fructose, and sucrose. And sucrose breaks down to glucose and fructose. The body treats fructose very differently than glucose. We'll explore the actions of fructose in Chapter 2.

Sugar Digestion and Absorption

Sugar digestion begins in the small intestine. (While it is true that digestion of carbohydrates begins in the mouth, only complex carbohydrates begin to be broken down by salivary amylase in the mouth.) The disaccharides (maltose, lactose and sucrose) are broken down into their component sugars (glucose, fructose, and galactose) at the brush border of the small intestine for absorption.

These resulting monosaccharides, glucose, fructose, and galactose, are absorbed in the small intestine and sent to the liver. The fate of fructose will be discussed in Chapter 2. Galactose metabolism is less significant as most of us ingest only small amounts each day, primarily from dairy products. In the liver, some glucose is converted to glycogen, the storage form of carbohydrates for later use. The remainder is released into the bloodstream, resulting in an increase in blood sugar levels after eating a meal or snack containing carbohydrates or sugar. The rate of rise in blood sugar levels depends on the amount of carbohydrate consumed and the glycemic index or load of that food, which I will discuss in Chapter 3 (7).

Blood Sugar Regulation

The regulator that determines how the body deals with glucose is insulin, a hormone secreted by the pancreatic beta-cells. The level of insulin that is produced increases with the glycemic load of the meal. Insulin performs the dual functions of sending glucose into your body cells as fuel and signaling the body to store fat. Blood glucose levels reach their peak anywhere from 30 minutes to 90 minutes after a meal. The glycemic load of the meal is the main determinant of how fast and high blood sugar levels rise.

CHAPTER 2: FRUCTOSE AND HIGH FRUCTOSE CORN SYRUP

Before really delving into the negative health effects of sugar, a discussion of fructose is in order. More and more research shows that the negative health effects of sugar are at least somewhat attributable to fructose. There has been much vigorous debate about whether high fructose corn syrup (HFCS) is worse than sugar, and by now many people believe it to be worse than sugar. I suspect table sugar and HFCS are just about equally as detrimental to health as they both break down similarly in the body. I do have concerns about the process of producing high fructose corn syrup - from the genetic modification of corn to the use of the toxic pesticides roundup and atrazine in the production of corn (8). But that is a topic for another day.

Let's start by examining what HFCS syrup actually is. Michael Pollan describes the process of making HFCS well in his book, *The Omnivore's Dilemma*. The starch from corn is broken down to glucose using enzymes. Fructose tastes sweeter than glucose, and for this reason, additional enzymes are used to convert glucose to fructose to yield a syrup that is 55% fructose, 42% glucose, and 3% other sugars. As a result, the sweetness of HFCS is about the same as that of table sugar (sucrose). The surplus of corn grown causes HFCS, despite all the steps required to produce it, to be a cheaper sweetener than table sugar (9).

When ingested, the glucose from table sugar and HFCS is absorbed into the bloodstream and raises blood glucose levels. This rise in blood glucose levels prompts the pancreas to secrete insulin. As discussed previously, insulin triggers the body to store excess glucose as fat. Fructose, on the other hand, goes straight to the liver and has virtually no effect on blood glucose levels. For this reason, fructose is often used in diabetic products to promote better blood sugar regulation and prevent the insulin spikes that lead to fat storage that occur when glucose is ingested (7). For comparison, the glycemic index (to be discussed in Chapter 3) of fructose is 22, with pure glucose as a reference set at 100. Briefly, the higher the glycemic index, the higher and faster your blood glucose level rises. Given the low glycemic index of fructose, the thought has been that fructose is beneficial to use as a sweetener in diabetic products, for example, since it minimally affects blood sugar levels. Unfortunately, fructose has the negative health effects of increasing abdominal fat storage, triglycerides levels, and blood sugar and cholesterol levels.

There have been multiple animal studies investigating the effects of fructose on health, but fewer human studies. One striking study compared the effects of drinking one liter of regular cola (sweetened with sucrose) versus semi-skim milk versus diet soda versus water every day in 47 overweight subjects for six months. The regular cola group had a significant increase in accumulation of visceral abdominal fat and liver fat, a 32% increase in triglyceride levels and an 11% increase in total cholesterol. There was no significant change in these parameters in the other beverage groups. The semi-skim milk used in this study supplied the same number of calories as the regular cola, but milk contains no fructose. The calorie content of milk comes from protein, lactose (which remember breaks down to glucose and galactose), and some fat. While not completely conclusive, based on other study results showing similar negative effects, the authors suggest that the fructose content of the regular soda may be responsible for the soda's negative effects. The authors note that average regular soda consumption in the US is 0.5 liters per day and much higher in other groups including young American men aged 12 to 29 who drink an average of 1.8 liters of soda daily (10)!

Further research points to fructose not only increasing triglycerides and abdominal fat, but also decreasing insulin sensitivity and promoting the accumulation of liver fat to the point of the development of non-alcoholic fatty liver disease (NAFLD) (11). In my practice, I have seen the reversal of fatty liver in a female client in her late 20s, who was obese and eating a high sugar and refined carbohydrate diet when we met. After she cut out sugar and followed a high protein and carbohydrate-controlled eating plan, she was able to lose more than 40 pounds and reverse the fatty liver. So for all the clinicians out there, when you have a patient with fatty liver, consider sugar (specifically fructose) as an underlying cause.

Another interesting study examined the effects of moderate amounts of fructose on insulin resistance and sensitivity. Nine healthy men ages 21-25 participated in this double-blind randomized cross-over trial. The participants consumed 600 mL daily (as three 200 mL beverages) of each of the following four beverages for three weeks at a time (40 grams fructose, 80 grams fructose, 80 grams glucose, 80 grams sucrose). The 80-gram fructose group showed signs of insulin resistance though this was not observed in the 40-gram fructose or glucose or sucrose group. In addition, both fructose groups and the sucrose group had statistically significantly higher total cholesterol and LDL cholesterol levels as compared to the glucose group. The authors note that fructose is quickly broken down in the liver into intermediates involved in the fat synthesis pathway, and this is likely how fructose effects cholesterol levels (12). Interesting here to note that sugar, not fat, is actually raising cholesterol levels.

Not all of the research on fructose is as conclusive. If you do a literature search, you will find articles disputing the idea that drinking sugar-sweetened beverages with fructose leads to abdominal visceral fat and elevated blood pressure. One particular article is entitled "Consumption of sucrose and high-fructose corn syrup does not increase liver fat or ectopic fat deposition in muscles." One of its authors has received consulting fees from the Corn Refiners Association, Pepsico, Kraft foods, and Weight Watchers (13). A second article disputes the idea that fructose increases the risk of high blood pressure (14). The authors had received funding from Coca-Cola.

Added sugars are not the only source of fructose. Fruit also contains a significant amount of naturally occurring fructose along with glucose and sucrose in varying proportions. In most fruit, the fructose content is similar or higher than the glucose content. See the chart to compare the amount of fructose in fruit to the amount obtained from foods and beverages with added sugars. The data presented in the table includes fructose and glucose that are a part of sucrose in food. Note that sugar-sweetened beverages like coke have the highest fructose content. Three oreo cookies have the same sugar breakdown as a banana, each with 7 grams of fructose and glucose. The banana, unlike the oreos, has nutritional value with significant amounts of potassium, vitamin C, and folate (15). As I will address in Chapter 8, evaluating your intake of natural sugar is important too, but the first steps are limiting sugar-sweetened beverages and desserts that lack any nutritional value in addition to their detrimental high sugar content.

Fructose and Glucose Content of Common Foods

Food/Beverage	Serving Size	Fructose (grams)	Glucose (grams)
Coke	12 oz.	22	16
Coke	32 oz.	60	43
Power bar	1 bar	11	8
Oreo cookies	3 cookies	7	7
Honey	1 tablespoon	9	8
Agave nectar	1 tablespoon	12	3
Banana	1 medium	7	7
Raspberries	1 cup	3	2
Blueberries	1 cup	7	7
Strawberries	1 cup	4	4
Apple	1 medium	13	6
Orange	1 medium	6	6
Peach	1 medium	6.5	6
Watermelon	1 cup	6	3
Cherries	1 cup	7	9

Data from USDA Food and Nutrient Database (15).

CHAPTER 3: GLYCEMIC INDEX AND GLYCEMIC LOAD

The glycemic index is a number assigned to foods with carbohydrates. It measures how much and how fast a particular food raises your blood sugar. Foods with a high glycemic index, which tend to be sugar-sweetened desserts, breakfast cereals, soda, and fruit juice, will raise your blood sugar quickly and to a higher level than low glycemic index foods like plain yogurt and low sugar fruits like raspberries and strawberries. These rapid blood sugar spikes lead to insulin spikes that promote fat storage by your body and leave you on a roller coaster of energy highs and lows throughout the day.

Glycemic index values are available in tables and on sites like glycemicindex.com (16), which is a collection of glycemic index values from a variety of research articles. In these studies, subjects were given a portion of a particular food to equal 25 or 50 grams of carbohydrate. The subjects' blood sugar was then measured over the following 2 hours after eating that food. The area under the glucose curve is then measured. That number is then expressed as a percentage of the area under the curve for pure glucose or white bread.

Whether glucose or white bread is used a standard, the glycemic index is set at 100. Thus the glycemic index of a food is a based on the blood sugar response elicited in a group of real people as compared to the blood sugar response to white bread or pure glucose. All the glycemic index data presented here used glucose as a standard.

Since the glycemic index is based on a 25 or 50-gram portion of carbohydrates in each food, the serving sizes vary considerably. For example, in order to obtain 50 grams of carbohydrates from carrots, you would need to eat 7 large carrots, which is much more than most people would eat at one time. The glycemic load, on the other hand, takes into account the serving size in determining the effect on blood sugar. Thus the glycemic load provides a more reliable measure of how a particular food will actually affect blood sugar when eaten in a normal-sized portion. Unlike the glycemic index that has to be measured experimentally, the glycemic load is a calculated value utilizing the glycemic index and the grams of carbohydrate in a particular food. To calculate the glycemic load, multiply the grams of carbohydrate in the serving size and divide by 100 (16). Factors that affect the glycemic index or load for a particular food include the protein, fat, and fiber content (7). Generally, the higher in fat, protein, and/or fiber the food is, the lower the glycemic index or load. This is because fat, protein, and fiber slow down the release of sugar into the bloodstream.

$$\text{Glycemic Load} = \frac{\text{Glycemic Index} * \text{grams of carbohydrate in serving size}}{100}$$

Since the glycemic index is a measured value based on the glucose response of research subjects, numbers will vary depending on what table or research article you consult. All glycemic index and load values presented here were determined using pure glucose as a standard. The University of Sydney advises an average glycemic index for your daily diet to be 45 or less (16). While an average glycemic index for a whole day of eating is not easy to calculate, the bottom line is that you always want to choose foods with lower glycemic index and load. Generally foods with larger amounts of added sugar and refined carbohydrates such as candy, sodas, and breakfast cereals will have the highest glycemic index values. The following chart lists common carbohydrate-containing foods in order of descending glycemic index. You notice that foods like Clif Bars, Power Bars, and Grape-nuts that many people consider healthy have a very high glycemic index. Based on the high glycemic index, these foods are best avoided. It's also interesting to note that, among the sweets on this list, the items with the lowest glycemic load are regular, full-fat ice cream and dark chocolate.

Glycemic Index and Load of Common Foods

Food/Beverage	Glycemic Index	Serving Size	Glycemic Load
Clif bar	101	1 bar	42
Powerbar	83	1 bar	37
Jellybeans	80	10 large	21
Cornflakes	80	1 cup	19
Grape-nuts	75	1/2 cup	33
Pop tart	70	1 package	25
Skittles	70	1 fun size package	13
Special K	69	1 cup	16
Kashi Whole grain puffs	65	1 cup	10
Coke	63	12 oz.	25
Banana	62	1 medium	17
Orange juice	50	8 oz.	13
Milk Chocolate	49	1.4 oz. (40g)	12
Ice cream, low-fat	47	1/2 cup	10
Twix	44	2 bars	15
Betty crocker vanilla cake with frosting	42	1/10 cake mix pkg + 2 tbsp frosting	24
Apple	39	1 medium	10
All-bran cereal	38	1 cup	17
Ice cream, regular	36	1/2 cup	6
Low-fat fruit-flavored yogurt	33	1 cup	14
Dark Chocolate	23	1.4 oz. (40g)	6
Plain whole milk yogurt	11	1 cup	1

Carbohydrate content used to calculate glycemic load from manufacturer's websites (current as of June 2013) and USDA Food and Nutrient Database (15). Glycemic index values from glycemic index.com (16) and international glycemic index tables (17).

PART 1 KEY POINTS

1. The main forms of sugar found in foods are sucrose, glucose, and fructose. Sucrose breaks down in the body to glucose and fructose.

2. Fructose is found in table sugar and most other added sugar sources such as HFCS, honey, maple syrup, molasses, rapadura, and fruit, and occurs in high levels in agave nectar.

3. Fructose may promote the storage of belly fat, fat around the organs, insulin resistance, and increase triglycerides and cholesterol levels.

4. The glycemic index and load are measures of how much a particular food raises your blood sugar. The glycemic index tells you the quality of the carbohydrate. The glycemic load is calculated from the glycemic index and takes into account the quality and quantity of carbohydrate ingested. The glycemic load is a better indicator than glycemic index of blood sugar response.

5. Choose lower glycemic index and load foods and always pair carbohydrate-containing foods with protein and healthy fats to keep blood sugar levels steady. The majority of foods you eat should have glycemic index of 45 or lower.

Part 2: Why Sugar Isn't So Sweet: The Health Hazards of Sugar

CHAPTER 4: IS SUGAR MAKING YOU GAIN WEIGHT?

It's a natural assumption to conclude that eating fat translates into fat on your body. Our bodies don't work quite so simply, as your body is capable of converting excess sugar and carbohydrates to fat as well. The inaccurate assumption that eating fat makes you fat has spawned the ongoing nutrition recommendations to focus on limiting fat in the diet, instead of the real culprit – sugar. There are a variety of political and financial interests that have influenced these recommendations. The sales of soda, sports drinks, other sugar-sweetened beverages, desserts, and sweetened yogurts and cereals are big business in the US. Large food companies with deep pockets tend to have considerable power in influencing health recommendations.

The other inaccurate assumption is the idea that calorie counting is the only thing that matters. I often hear the quote from healthcare professionals that "calories in and calories out. It's a simple equation. If you burn more calories than you take in, you'll lose weight." I find this statement so exasperating, because our bodies are highly complex machines with important hormones like insulin and thyroid hormones that govern metabolism, weight, fat burning, and fat storage. The human body is complicated and dynamic, and the cause of weight gain cannot be reduced to a simple equation.

Sugar and excess carbohydrates tend to result in weight gain through the actions of insulin. The high carbohydrate and low-fat diet of the 1980s famously failed at helping people achieve lasting weight loss. This made way for the more successful reduced carbohydrate diets that work via the reduction of insulin levels. Smaller amounts of total carbohydrates and sugar result in lower levels of insulin being released by the pancreas in order to regulate blood sugar levels. Because one of the signals insulin provides to the body is to store fat, reducing carbohydrates effectively turns down the signal to store fat. As discussed in Chapter 2, fructose may also play a role in weight gain by decreasing insulin sensitivity and promoting fat storage around the belly (18). I have had clients lose up to 10 pounds in the first week after quitting a 32-oz. or more daily soda habit along with a reduction in sugar and refined carbohydrates and an increase in protein.

CHAPTER 5: SUGAR AND DIABETES, METABOLIC SYNDROME, AND HEART DISEASE

Now I really want to get down to the nitty gritty research on the negative health effects of sugar to show that there is convincing evidence for the hazards of sugar. Allow me to start with this quote from a 2013 article in *Current Opinion in Lipidology* (19), in which the authors conclude that "the accumulating epidemiological evidence, direct clinical evidence, and the evidence suggesting plausible mechanisms support a role for sugar in the epidemics of metabolic syndrome, cardiovascular disease, and type II diabetes." I would use even stronger language based on the patterns I see again and again in the eating habits of those with diabetes and heart disease. While not scientific, actual experience talking to people about their daily diet provides powerful insight. I believe excess sugar and refined carbohydrates intake to be at the root of many of the worst health problems out there today. There are of course other factors like lack of fruits and vegetables and lack of exercise, but I consider sugar the primary problem, when you consider an average daily sugar intake of 94 grams or about 23 teaspoons in the US (2).

We're going to explore the research on how sugar, fructose, glycemic index and load, and refined carbohydrate intake may affect risk of diabetes, cardiovascular disease, metabolic syndrome, and cancer development and progression. The intent here is not to provide an exhaustive analysis of the research linking sugar and these health conditions, but to give you an overview of the research and proposed mechanisms by which sugar increases risk of disease. The research is not yet conclusive. To wait until it is, when the effect of limiting sugar is only positive and causes no harm, is a risk that I wouldn't advise taking.

Type 2 Diabetes

First of all, Type 2 diabetes should not be confused with type 1 diabetes, also known as childhood diabetes, in which an autoimmune reaction destroys the beta-cells in the pancreas, so that the pancreas no longer produces insulin. With insulin no longer being produced, blood sugar remains very high as the glucose has no way to get into the cells of the body to be used for energy. People with type 1 diabetes require insulin injections to regulate blood sugar.

Let's first discuss the process of development of type 2, or adult onset, diabetes. The general progression of type 2 diabetes is the onset of insulin resistance, which proceeds to pre-diabetes and finally diabetes. In insulin resistance, insulin becomes less effective at getting glucose into the cells of the body therefore becoming less able to regulate blood sugar levels. As insulin resistance progresses, pre-diabetes results because the cells of the body have become resistant to the actions of insulin. This causes glucose to remain in the blood longer, and blood glucose remains elevated for longer periods of time. In pre-diabetes, fasting blood glucose levels are between 100-125 mg/dL, as compared to less than 100 mg/dL in healthy folks. The other diagnostic criteria include Hemoglobin A1C of 5.7-6.4% or 2-hour post-prandial blood glucose of 140-199 mg/dL. Pre-diabetes may then progress to diabetes. Diabetes is diagnosed based on having at least one of the following 4 criteria. A positive test needs to be confirmed on another day in order to confirm the diagnosis:

o   Hemoglobin A1C of 6.5% or higher.

o   Fasting blood glucose levels over 125 mg/dL
o   Blood glucose of 200 mg/dL or higher 2 hours after drinking a sugar solution containing 75 grams glucose, known as an oral glucose tolerance test.
o   Random blood glucose reading of 200 mg/dL or higher along with diabetes symptoms (20).

All of these diagnostic criteria are indicators of elevated blood glucose levels. Part of the process in the development of diabetes is the ability of the pancreas to compensate for the insulin resistance. As the cells of the body become more and more resistant to the actions of insulin, the pancreas compensates by pumping out more insulin. Over time, the exhausted pancreas is no longer able to keep up with insulin demand and eventually starts producing less and less insulin. It is often then that a diabetic needs to start insulin injections (21).

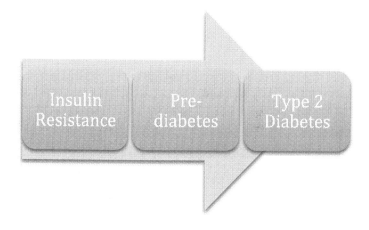

The consequences of having diabetes with frequently elevated blood glucose are quite devastating. The elevated glucose damages blood vessels throughout the body, which may lead to declines in vision, kidney function and blood circulation, as well as neuropathy (damage to the nerves), heart disease, and diabetic ulcers. Diabetic ulcers or wounds, commonly found on the feet, are a result of decreased circulation and inadequate blood flow and delivery of nutrients for healing. A simple way of thinking about how elevated blood sugar damages your body is to think of sugar crystals in your blood stream making tiny little scratches and damaging structures throughout the body. The more sugar crystals roaming around in the bloodstream, the more damage results. In extreme cases, uncontrolled diabetes can lead to blindness, kidney failure necessitating dialysis, and amputations of limbs due to infection of non-healing wounds (21). Nobody wants any of these things to happen!

Now that I've covered the development and adverse effects of diabetes, I need to get back to the central and hotly debated question as to whether sugar *causes* diabetes or not. From a logical standpoint, given the physiology of diabetes development, it stands to reason that excess carbohydrates and sugar should play a major role in the development of diabetes, but this is not an accepted mechanism by the "experts," including the American Diabetes Association. The American Diabetes Association actually calls it a "myth" that eating too much sugar causes diabetes, though they do concede that drinking sugar-sweetened beverages increases risk of diabetes (22). I'm not sure what aspect of sugar-sweetened beverages they think is causing the diabetes if it's not the sugar!

Before we dive into the research, let's talk about why the research is convincing, but not completely conclusive. The research is lacking partly because the large studies needed are expensive and take a long time to conduct. In addition, diabetes generally takes many years to develop, and assessing someone's diet at one point in time (as many studies do) may not accurately assess his or her average intake over the time period of the study.

Now let's look at the research that has been done. In a 2010 meta-analysis of studies looking at risk for diabetes and metabolic syndrome with sugar-sweetened beverage intake, people with the highest intakes of sugar-sweetened beverages had a 26% higher risk of developing type 2 diabetes and a 20% higher risk of developing metabolic syndrome as compared to people with the lowest intake of sugar-sweetened beverages. I will not belabor this point, but suffice it to say that all the studies included in the meta-analysis except for one showed an increased risk for type 2 diabetes with increasing sugar-sweetened beverage consumption. This included a study in which people that drank more than one sugar-sweetened beverage daily had an 83% higher risk for type 2 diabetes as compared to those who consumed less than 1 per month (23). Pretty striking!

Dr. Robert Lustig, a Pediatric Endocrinologist at the University of California-San Francisco, is best known for his lecture entitled "Sugar: The Bitter Truth," and his book *Fat Chance: Beating the Odds against Sugar, Processed Food, Obesity, and Disease.* There, he and his and colleagues established a relationship between sugar availability and diabetes risk in countries throughout the world. Using their model, they found that every 150 calories/person/day increase in sugar availability was associated with a 1.1% increased risk for diabetes. While they examined other parts of the food supply, they were unable to find any associations with diabetes risk other than sugar. Sugar's impact was independent of physical activity level and overweight or obesity. Lustig et al note that sugar, especially fructose, increases risk for metabolic syndrome and diabetes independent of obesity. The authors point out that there are obese people with totally normal blood sugar and insulin regulation and that up to 40% (yes 40%!!) of normal weight people exhibit some of the characteristics of metabolic syndrome (24). I discuss metabolic syndrome coming up but the five attributes involved in metabolic syndrome are increased waist circumference due to belly fat accumulation, elevated triglycerides, blood pressure, and fasting blood glucose, and low level of high density lipoprotein (HDL) cholesterol.

The research shows that sugar-sweetened beverages increase the risk for insulin resistance and type 2 diabetes. While I feel pretty comfortable making the leap that higher intakes of sugar from cookies, cakes, sweets, yogurts, etc. play a role in diabetes development, the research hasn't been quite as clear on this point. While I know that this all sounds ominous, the beauty of it is that for many people these conditions are reversible. Cutting out the soda, the sweetened iced teas, and sports drinks and overall sugar intake are the first and most high impact steps to reducing and even reversing diabetes or pre-diabetes in the earlier stages. If you have type 2 diabetes and are already dependent on insulin injections, cutting your sugar intake can help you manage your blood sugar levels and prevent the complications of diabetes.

Cardiovascular Disease

While many people won't experience the debilitating and terrible side effects of diabetes, most people with diabetes will experience varying degrees of damage to their body. Diabetics have higher rates of heart disease than the general population, pointing to the fact that damage from excessive sugar intake, as opposed to fat, is a very real cause of heart disease. According to the American Diabetes Association, 2 out of 3 people with diabetes will die from heart disease or a stroke (25).

In the research, higher intakes of sugar-sweetened beverages like soda and sweetened juices and teas increase risk factors, not only for type 2 diabetes, but also cardiovascular disease. Research from data in the Nurse's Health Study cites a 28-44% increase in hypertension (high blood pressure) with high intakes of sugar-sweetened beverages. In addition, the Framingham study, most noted for establishing the link between cholesterol and heart disease, noted a 20% increase in hypertension in people who drank more than 1 sweetened soft drink daily as compared to those who never drank sweetened soft drinks (14). Dr. Lustig attributes the blood pressure raising effects of sugar to fructose, as fructose increases levels of uric acid, which raises blood pressure (18).

Not only is sugar able to increase blood pressure, but it may also increase cholesterol levels as seen in the study of nine young men who drank fructose, sucrose or glucose-sweetened beverages. The fructose and sucrose-sweetened drinks resulted in higher total and LDL cholesterol levels, though this was not observed when the subjects drank the glucose-sweetened beverage. This underscores the fact that fructose is responsible for the increase in total and LDL cholesterol levels, since the sucrose breaks down into fructose and glucose. Only the beverage that didn't contain any fructose did not have a negative impact on cholesterol levels (12).

Another vivid example of the role that sugar plays in the development of heart disease is dental health. In recent years, research has clearly shown a correlation between periodontal disease and heart disease risk. The American Heart Disease refutes the notion that dental problems actually cause an increase in heart disease risk (26). Instead, according to Spreadbury et al, the data suggest that carbohydrate-dense foods such as added sugars change the species of bacteria present in the mouth and small intestine to strains that produce more inflammation. The change to more inflammatory bacterial strains in the mouth results in tooth decay and periodontal disease, while inflammatory bacterial strains in the intestine may lead to atherosclerosis and heart disease (27).

Metabolic Syndrome

Metabolic syndrome really encompasses markers of the three disease states we just discussed – type 2 diabetes, heart disease, and overweight/obesity. Metabolic syndrome is truly a syndrome in that people will present with a constellation of symptoms. There are 5 criteria used in diagnosing metabolic syndrome. Three of the 5 criteria must be present for a diagnosis of metabolic syndrome. The criteria include the following:

1. Waist circumference greater than 35 inches for women and greater than 40 inches for men.
2. Triglycerides of 150 mg/dL or higher.
3. HDL cholesterol less than 50 mg/dL in women and less than 40 mg/dL in men.
4. Systolic blood pressure 130 mm Hg or higher or diastolic blood pressure of 85 mm Hg or higher.
5. Fasting blood glucose of 100 mg/dL or higher (28).

As discussed previously, there is research to support the role of sugar, especially fructose, in the development of abdominal weight gain, elevated triglycerides, elevated blood pressure, and elevated fasting blood sugar. Taken together, sugar provides the perfect storm for the development of metabolic syndrome. It's important to note that people do not have to be overweight or obese to be diagnosed with metabolic syndrome, though many obese people have metabolic syndrome. You can be thin or overweight and have metabolic syndrome. Being overweight is not a certain indicator of metabolic syndrome. Often people become overweight as a result of their sugar intake, which only facilitates development of the other attributes of metabolic syndrome (18).

CHAPTER 6: SUGAR AND CANCER RISK AND PROGRESSION

Many of you will have heard the statistics that 1 in every 2 men and 1 in every 3 women will be diagnosed with cancer in their lifetime (29). Some of these cancers will be curable, while others will lead to eventual death. I think it's easy when you're young to think that cancer is something that isn't going to happen to you if you're outwardly healthy. Or I often hear the exasperated exclamation "Everything causes cancer!" What I will tell you is that in my work with cancer patients, most people who have cancer would gladly change their diet if it meant they wouldn't have cancer. If you have cancer, there is nothing you wouldn't do to get rid of it, and at this point the treatment with surgery, chemotherapy, and radiation is something I wouldn't wish on anyone. The best thing you can do is to use everything in your power to prevent yourself from getting cancer. While there are always genetic and environmental causes of cancer, more than half of all cancers could be prevented with appropriate diet and lifestyle choices, according to the American Cancer Society (30).

So let's explore the research on sugar and cancer risk. One way that sugar may play a role in the development of cancer is partially through the promotion of overweight and obesity. According to the World Research Fund's 2nd Expert Report, there is convincing evidence that body fatness increases risk for esophageal, colorectal, pancreatic, endometrial, kidney, and postmenopausal breast cancer (31). As discussed earlier, higher sugar and refined carbohydrate intake can be a major cause of overweight and obesity.

In addition, according to a joint opinion released by the American Diabetes Association and the American Cancer Society, having diabetes (primarily type 2 diabetes) is associated with an increased risk for liver, pancreatic, endometrial colorectal, breast, and bladder cancer. The proposed mechanisms are elevated insulin levels, elevated blood sugar, and inflammation, all of which may promote the development of cancer (32).

I am presenting a sampling of the relevant studies showing the effect of higher sugar, glycemic index or glycemic load, added sugar or total carbohydrate intake on breast, endometrial, prostate cancer, and colon cancer risk and progression. I also outline studies linking insulin levels and cancer risk, since insulin levels are so directly influenced by sugar and carbohydrate intake.

Breast Cancer

Breast cancer is the most common type of cancer among women in the United States. Obesity is a known risk factor for post-menopausal breast cancer, and one of the mechanisms for this increased risk is related to the excess estrogen produced in the fat tissue. In addition, animal and cell culture studies have demonstrated that insulin increases cell proliferation and tumor cell growth. Obesity has been linked to chronically high levels of insulin. Thus we have high estrogen and high insulin levels both as promoters of breast cancer development. Being overweight increases total estrogen production in the fat tissue, and being overweight is often a result of excess sugar intake as discussed in Chapter 4. Elevated insulin levels are a sign of insulin resistance, also often a consequence of excess sugar intake.

In a prospective case-cohort study as part of the Women's Health Initiative, post-menopausal women (who were not using hormone therapy) with the highest insulin levels had a 2.4-fold increased risk of breast cancer (33). These results were confirmed in another analysis of the Women's Health Initiative data, in which elevated insulin levels were associated with 2 to 3-fold increased risk of breast cancer (regardless of whether or not they used hormone therapy), but elevated glucose levels were not associated with an increased risk. Insulin is likely to play a more direct role in cancer development as opposed to blood glucose levels, but it's important to note that blood glucose levels directly affect insulin levels and vice versa (34).

While elevated insulin levels seem to clearly increase risk for post-menopausal breast cancer, other research has not been able to establish a link between glycemic index, glycemic load, added sugar, or total carbohydrate intake, and breast cancer risk (35). I suspect this is related to the fact that likely very few women in these studies have a very low glycemic or low carbohydrate diet, since there just isn't a big segment of the US population with really low sugar or carbohydrate intake. For example, the lowest level of added sugar intake in this study was considered 18 grams or less of added sugar. While this is significantly lower than the average American's sugar intake, it's not that low! It's very difficult to assess the beneficial effect of a diet very low in added sugar when there are so few people who consume such a diet.

Endometrial Cancer

Another type of cancer that plagues women is endometrial cancer, which is cancer of the uterine ling. In a case-control study of 822 women using interview and food frequency questionnaire, women with highest added sugar intake or more than 34.2 grams (per 1000 calories) had an 84% increased risk for endometrial cancer compared to women in the lowest category of added sugar intake or less than 16.3 grams (per 1000 calories). If you assume a 2000 calorie per day diet, even an added sugar intake under 33 grams per day was beneficial in reducing risk of endometrial cancer. I would consider 33 grams of added sugar too much to be consuming on a daily basis, but I will discuss that further in chapter 7. This increased risk of cancer with higher added sugar intake was independent of BMI, meaning that it wasn't simply that the excess sugar was causing women to be overweight, which increased their risk for endometrial cancer. It seems to be the sugar itself that is having the negative effect. The authors hypothesize that insulin may directly promote tumor growth. Alternatively, elevated insulin levels are know to increase the production of androgens (including testosterone), which leads to lack of ovulation and low progesterone and often lack of menstruation, which is known to increase endometrial cancer risk. High levels of estrogen accompanied by low progesterone may promote endometrial cancer as well (36).

Prostate cancer
Diabetics have a lower risk of prostate cancer compared to non-diabetics, according the American Diabetes Association (32). Prostate cancer is the only type of cancer in which this association has been observed. On the contrary, other evidence points to carbohydrate and sugar intake as drivers of prostate cancer risk and progression. In a 2012 Swedish study, higher intakes of certain types of refined carbohydrates including cakes and biscuits and low fiber cereals were associated with increased risk for prostate cancer. Higher intakes of sugar-sweetened beverages were also associated with an increased risk of symptomatic prostate cancer (37). In another study looking at prostate cancer progression, the authors concluded that replacing 10% of calorie intake from carbohydrate with vegetable fat was associated with a lower risk of lethal prostate cancer and all cause mortality underscoring the detrimental effects of excess carbohydrates, with fat actually showing a benefit (38). Further research has been underway at Duke University investigating whether low carbohydrate ketogenic diets in mice may help reduce prostate cancer progression (39). A

ketogenic diet is one that is very low in carbohydrates and higher in fat with a moderate amount of protein. In following a ketogenic diet, the body breaks down fat for energy, which produces ketones that are burned for energy instead of carbohydrates.

Colon Cancer

There is emerging research looking at the impact of sugar on the risk and progression of colon cancer. By progression, I mean once a person has colon cancer, how does their intake of sugar affect their rate of recurrence (the cancer coming back) and how long they live.

In a case-control study of a Scottish cohort, higher intakes of sugar-sweetened beverages and high-energy snack foods were associated with increased risk of colorectal cancer. High-energy snack foods were defined as high sugar and high fat foods like desserts, chips, chocolate, and nuts. It's hard to draw too many conclusions from the high energy snacks group, since sugar and fat were lumped together. It's unclear whether the increased risk is due to the sugar, fat, or combination of the two. Based on the fact that sugar-sweetened beverages seem to increase colorectal cancer risk, I would suspect sugar is responsible for at least part of this increased risk (40).

An interesting study, from the Journal of the National Cancer Institute, looked at the effect of glycemic index, glycemic load, fructose, and total carbohydrate intake on cancer progression in patients with stage III colon cancer. This large study of 1011 colon cancer patients found that patients with the highest glycemic load diet (as compared to the group with the lowest glycemic load diet) had highest risk of colon cancer recurrence and death. In addition, higher total fructose intake resulted in shorter recurrence-free survival indicating that higher fructose intake may increase risk for recurrence. Higher total carbohydrate intake was correlated with increased risk of death from any cause as well as recurrence of colon cancer. No significant differences were found for glycemic index. This is very striking evidence that after diagnosis of colon cancer, reducing sugar intake is important to help prevent cancer recurrence and in order to live longer (41).

The Bottom Line

While I have only presented a small portion of research showing an impact of sugar intake and sugar-related variables (glycemic index and load, insulin, total carbohydrate, added sugar) on cancer risk, I consider the evidence striking given few people think of sugar intake as a risk factor for cancer. Cancer patients often choose to cut out sugar, because "I heard that sugar feeds cancer." I have seen this notion quickly squashed by well-meaning healthcare providers who fear that cancer patients, who are often at risk of malnutrition, may further increase the likelihood they will become malnourished if they cut out sugar. However, the evidence does suggest that sugar may play a role in driving cancer development and progression. Antioxidant-rich fruits and vegetables are usually the first food items that people think of when it comes to cancer prevention, but increasing these beneficial items without cutting your sugar intake may leave you at a continued risk for cancer.

PART 2 KEY POINTS

1. Sugar promotes weight gain due to the glucose, which increase insulin levels, promoting fat storage. The fructose component of sugar also promotes belly fat accumulation.

2. Higher sugar intake and availability, especially from sugar-sweetened beverages increases risk of type 2 diabetes through the progression from insulin resistance to pre-diabetes to diabetes.

3. Higher intakes of sugar and sugar-sweetened beverages may increase risk for high blood pressure and elevated total and LDL cholesterol levels, all markers of cardiovascular disease.

4. Metabolic Syndrome is characterized by 3 of the following 5 characteristics: increased waist circumference, elevated triglycerides, low HDL, high blood pressure, and elevated fasting blood glucose. All of these, with the exception of low HDL, can be a consequence of excess sugar intake.

5. Elevated insulin levels have been associated with increased risk of breast cancer, while higher added sugar intake may increase endometrial cancer risk. Sugar-sweetened beverages and desserts may play a role in the development of prostate cancer. Higher sugar-sweetened beverage intake is associated with higher risk of colon cancer. Colon cancer may progress more quickly with higher fructose and total carbohydrate intake and higher glycemic load diet.

6. You don't have to be overweight or obese to be at increased risk for these health problems. Excess sugar intake may promote the development of diabetes, cardiovascular disease, metabolic syndrome, and certain types of cancer all on its own.

Part 3: Kicking the Sugar Habit

CHAPTER 7: HOW MUCH SUGAR IS TOO MUCH?

The answer to the question of how much added sugar is too much is different depending on whom you ask. My answer is that your added sugar intake should be as low as possible. If you're currently taking in 50 grams of added sugar daily, then cutting down to 25 daily is a huge improvement. If your sugar intake is 25 grams, you should strive for even lower. Before addressing total added sugar intake in detail, allow me to summarize the recommendations from the US government and other major non-governmental health associations:

US Department of Agriculture (USDA) on Myplate.gov: "A small amount of empty calories is okay, but most people eat *far more* than is healthy. It is important to limit empty calories to the amount that fits your calorie and nutrient needs. You can lower your intake by eating and drinking foods and beverages containing empty calories *less often* or by decreasing the *amount* you eat or drink." The USDA also states the more active you are the more empty calories you can consume. The stated acceptable range for daily "empty calories" is stated as 120-330 calories per day for adults, with empty calories defined as calories from solid fats or added sugars (42). If empty calories were coming only from sugar, this is the equivalent 30-83 grams of added sugar daily!

Dietary Guidelines for All Americans: "Consume fewer foods with sodium (salt), saturated fats, *trans* fats, cholesterol, added sugars, and refined grains. Reduce intake of sugar-sweetened beverages." These guidelines give no specific recommendations on how much sugar is safe to consume (3).

American Cancer Society: "Limit your intake of sugar-sweetened beverages such as soft drinks, sports drinks, and fruit-flavored drinks. When you eat away from home, be especially mindful to choose food low in calories, fat, and added sugar, and avoid eating large portion sizes (43)." Again no specific recommendation on amount of sugar.

American Diabetes Association: "Save money by buying less soda, sweets and chips or other snack foods." For preventing diabetes, no specific guidelines on limiting sugar intake are provided (44).

American Heart Association (AHA): The AHA recommendation is no more than 25 grams of added sugar per day for women or about 6 teaspoons. For men, the AHA recommends no more than 36 grams of added sugar per day for men or about 9 teaspoons (45).

As you can see many of the top health organizations remain focused on the need to reduce fat and sodium in the diet with little specific guidance in reducing sugar. When specific guidelines are given, they do not go far enough. In my opinion our goal, as lofty as it may sound, is to have less than 10 grams of added sugar most days of the week. This is approximately equivalent to 2 teaspoons of maple syrup or 1 ½ teaspoons of honey daily. No added sugar is even better. There is no level of added sugar that is good for you or needed. Perhaps a couple times per week, you savor a special dessert with added sugar. If you do eat sweets every day, you are likely not enjoying them as much as you would if you only had them on special occasions or with special meals. Remember, it's not a party if it happens everyday.

Keep in mind that I'm referring to added sugars, not the naturally occurring sugars in fruit, which is where the majority of the sweetness you ingest should come from. Added sugar is not always easy to calculate, as "added sugar" is not an item that's listed on food labels.

Nutrition Facts

Serving Size 1 Cake (43g)
Servings Per Container 5

Amount Per Serving

Calories 200 Calories from Fat 90

	% Daily Value*
Total Fat 10g	15%
Saturated Fat 5g	25%
Trans Fat 0g	
Cholesterol 0mg	0%
Sodium 100mg	4%
Total Carbohydrate 26g	9%
Dietary Fiber 0g	0%
Sugars 19g	
Protein 1g	

Vitamin A 0%	•	Vitamin C 0%
Calcium 0%	•	Iron 2%

The arrows show the total carbohydrate and total sugar content on a food label. Added sugar is not listed on the label.

It can be difficult to figure out the added sugar content of foods, because many foods have natural sugar and added sugar. Luckily, I've done some of this math for you. Use the chart to determine the added sugar content of some common foods.

Total and Added Sugar Content of Common Foods

Food/Beverage	Serving Size	Total Sugar (grams)	Added Sugar (grams)
Coke	12 oz.	39	39
Coke	32 oz.	104	104
Instant oatmeal (sweetened)	1 packet	11	11
Fiber one bar	1 bar	9	9
Power bar	1 bar	25-29	25-29
Breyer's vanilla ice cream	½ cup	11	11
Breyer's cookies in cream ice cream	½ cup	12	12
Oreo cookies	3 cookies	13	13
Fruit flavored low-fat yogurt	1 cup	42	26
Plain nonfat yogurt	1 cup	19	0
Plain low-fat yogurt	1 cup	16	0
Plain whole milk yogurt	1 cup	11	0
Banana	1 medium	14	0
Raspberries	1 cup	5	0

Data from manufacturer's websites (current as of June 2013) and USDA Food and Nutrient Database (15).

A good example of the combination of natural sugar and added sugar is yogurt. (Another good example would be a dessert or beverage that contains natural sugar from the fruit as well as added sugar.) Yogurt has naturally occurring sugar in the form of lactose, so flavored and sweetened yogurts will have "sugars" listed on the label. Generally the lower the fat content of yogurt, the higher the naturally occurring lactose (milk sugar) content. One cup of full-fat plain yogurt has 11 grams of lactose, while nonfat plain yogurt has 19 grams lactose. You can use these numbers as a guideline when trying to figure out the added sugar content of your favorite yogurt. Subtract the total sugar content of plain yogurt (be sure to choose the right type – whole milk, non fat, or low-fat) from the total sugar content listed on the label. For example, if a low-fat flavored yogurt has 42 grams of sugar listed, 16 grams are natural sugars and the other 26 grams are added sugar. You can see that even eating one cup of flavored yogurt could put you above the AHA's lax sugar limits for women! I'm not intending to say that it's ok to eat as much natural sugar as you want, but reducing added sugar is the first step. Then you move on to make sure you're aren't overdoing the natural sugars either, which you will learn about in Chapter 8.

CHAPTER 8: CUTTING BACK ON SWEETS STEP BY STEP

One of the most frequent questions that I receive in my practice is "I'm constantly craving sugar. What do I do?" Many people report having a major sweet tooth, craving something sweet after most meals. We often crave what we eat regularly, so it's no surprise if you are used to having sweets after lunch and dinner every day that your body automatically craves them. It's almost a Pavlovian response. In the same way that a dog is trained to salivate with the ringing of a bell since the sound of the bell is associated with food, we associate the finishing of a meal with the desire for something sweet.

Sugar has an addictive quality to it. According to the research, sugar can interfere with the hormone leptin, which signals the body to feel full and satisfied. Therefore your appetite effectively increases when you eat sugar or drink sugar-sweetened beverages. It can also decrease dopamine signaling. Dopamine is a neurotransmitter involved in pleasure. When dopamine signaling is disrupted, you continue to seek more food in order to achieve the expected pleasure (18).

For most people, the most effective way to decrease your sugar cravings is to give them up for at least 1 week. This week will be hard for most but at the end of it, you will crave sweets less. For most people, the sweet cravings will never completely go away. These sweet cravings are evolutionary — a desire for sweets would lead humans to seek out foods with calories in order to provide sustenance. The types of sweet foods available to our hunter gatherer ancestors would have been fruits, not even as sweet as the fruit we have today, which has been bred for sweetness. In the current food environment where food is plentiful, this desire for sweets often leads us to overeat them. Limiting sweets requires discipline and being in tune with your body and noticing and celebrating the perceptible victories like weight loss and improved energy and mood. It also requires finding motivation in the imperceptible victories like improvement in health and reduction in disease risk that occur as a result of reducing your sugar intake.

As you work toward reducing your sugar intake, follow this step-by-step process, skipping any steps that are not relevant for you:

1. **Wean yourself off of all soda.** (If you don't drink soda, move on to step 2). Drinking your sweets especially in the form of soda is a recipe for weight gain, unstable energy levels, mood swings, and future disease. Soda is carbonated, colored sugar water and nothing more. Diet soda is not a valid alternative. The artificial sweeteners in diet soda taste so much sweeter than sugar that they serve only to exacerbate your sugar cravings and derange your body's reaction to carbohydrates. See Chapter 10 to learn more about the negative health effects of artificial sweeteners.

2. **Eliminate all other sweetened beverages.** This includes bottled teas, Kool-Aid, juices and smoothies with added sugar. I'm not referring to the naturally occurring sugar in foods like fruit at this point. This also needs to be considered, but comes along later in the process.

Now that you've eliminated many beverages from your life, what should you drink? Water is of course a great option, but for those that need flavor as well, try cucumber or lemon water or a sparkling water with a splash of 100% fruit juice like tart cherry or pomegranate juice. Green, black, white or herbal tea are other great options and are rich sources of antioxidants. Nettle tea is an especially healthy herbal tea due to its content of calcium and other beneficial vitamins and minerals. When you want a nutritious and flavorful beverage, try vegetable juice, such as carrot-celery-kale juice that is packed with beneficial nutrients and antioxidants. Check out the recipe section for ideas.

3. **Scale back on desserts.** As much as you might think you *need* ice cream or a cookie after dinner every night, you really don't *need* it. You *want* it. The sooner you are able to acknowledge that, the better. Often many of us want to throw an inner temper tantrum, when we realize that the things we look to for comfort or escape are not truly serving us. This is the case with desserts. They may feel so familiar and comfortable – especially the desserts of your youth if you had a happy childhood. It's important to find a way to have desserts be a special treat – best saved for special occasions.

4. **Limit non-dessert foods with added sugar.** Unfortunately, there are many foods that we don't think of as dessert or don't even think of as that particularly sweet that contain added sugar. Flavored yogurts, oatmeal, soy and almond milks, and even foods you don't think of as sweet like breads, crackers, pasta and barbecue sauces, ketchup, and even some sausages have added sugar. Make sure to read the ingredient list of the foods you are buying and look for sugar, high fructose corn syrup, evaporated cane juice, fructose, honey, maltose syrup, brown rice syrup, honey, and maple syrup in the ingredient list. Instead add fruit to plain yogurt. If you need more sweetness, add a little bit of honey. This small amount of honey will provide much less sugar than the added sugar content of sweetened yogurts. Same goes for oatmeal – sweeten it yourself or use fruit as the

sweetener. There is no reason that crackers or breads need to be sweet. Buy the unsweetened varieties. I even like to use tomato paste instead of ketchup. The tomatoes have plenty of natural sweetness.

5. **Make sure you aren't overeating foods with naturally occurring sugars.** These are the sugars that naturally occur in fruit, for example, or the naturally occurring lactose in milk. Eating foods with naturally occurring sugar is a great way to satisfy your sweet tooth, but it's really important not to go overboard. For example, fruit juice contains natural sugar from the fruit, but when you drink fruit juice in excess, it can lead to weight gain and problems with blood sugar regulation since it is a big source of sugar, albeit natural sugar. For example, one cup of orange juice has 21 grams of sugar with 10 grams of sucrose, 6 grams of fructose, and 5 grams of glucose (15). Fruit juice is best avoided, except for every now and then. Very dilute fruit juice is ok, as is a splash of 100% juice in sparkling water, but is best reserved for very hot days or after intense exercise. If it's a choice between drinking soda or fruit juice, then fruit juice wins.

Fruit has some really wonderful health benefits, but there is such a thing as eating too much fruit. Aim for 2-4 servings of fruit/day in order to receive the beneficial vitamins, minerals, and phytonutrients from fruit without going overboard on the sugar. If you are someone who tends to eat more fruit than vegetables, you need to shift that balance to more vegetables than fruit. Vegetables are generally much richer sources of vitamins and minerals than fruit, while being mostly devoid of sugar.

CHAPTER 9: MY TOP 10 TIPS FOR KICKING YOUR SUGAR HABIT

1. Never eat sweets on an empty stomach. This is a recipe for a "carb coma" - high blood sugar with an energy rush followed by an energy crash that leads to subsequent sugar cravings. Best case scenario is to avoid eating any sweets until after dinner. The earlier in the day you start eating sweets, the more likely it is that you'll continue to eat sweets throughout the day.

2. Eat more protein. Protein is the number one thing that will help you feel full and satisfied and therefore less likely to crave sweets. Protein when paired with carbohydrates also helps to keep blood sugar levels steadier and decreases the glycemic load of a meal by slowing absorption of glucose (from broken down carbohydrates or sugar) into the bloodstream. Protein-rich foods are meat, eggs, fish, beans, dairy, and nuts and seeds.

3. Brush your teeth after eating. Sometimes the sweetness of the toothpaste is enough and the act of brushing your teeth means that mealtime is over and can help you move on to other activities. Also, ice cream or a cookie just doesn't seem quite as appealing when you have a minty taste in your mouth.

4. Practice productive distraction. In other words, when you keep thinking about eating sweets, consciously decide to shift your focus to something else. Try having a cup of your favorite tea, reading a good book, hugging someone, or going for walk. Often, it's not the sweet that we really need, but instead a nurturing distraction from our everyday activities.

5. Avoid saboteurs. For many people, the workplace is the worst source of sabotage when trying to improve your eating. Clients, patients, or staff may bring in sweets or co-workers have candy jars at their desk. I have heard many stories from my clients whose co-workers give them a hard time for turning down the steady stream of sweets in the office in order to lose weight or get healthier. These positive behavior changes should be celebrated, but instead are unfortunately often chided by others who have more trouble making good choices. I'm not saying you should never have sweets at work. Eating a small piece of a dessert at a party on occasion is fine. It's the daily habit of indulgence that becomes problematic.

6. Don't keep any sweets at home. If you really want to be successful, making it harder to have sweets when you have a craving is important. If you have to get in your car and drive somewhere to get those cookies, it's less likely that you'll do it. You will have to get all of the members of your household on board for this one. Have naturally sweet foods on hand to help satisfy cravings.

7. Get enough sleep. I can't stress this one enough. It's not only more difficult to make good decisions when you're sleep deprived, but inadequate sleep is associated with decreases in levels of the hormone leptin, leading to decreased satiety and increases in ghrelin, which in turn increases appetite. Evidence also suggests a role for sleep deprivation in the development of obesity and type II diabetes. In a study comparing 5 hours versus 9 hours of sleep, the sleep deprived participants consumed significantly higher total calories daily especially in the evening and higher levels of total carbohydrate (46). Furthermore, in a small study done at the University of Chicago, seven people were either allowed 4.5 hours or 8.5 hours in bed with controlled calorie intake and physical activity for 4 days. The lesser sleep amount resulted in more insulin resistance within the fat cells. Based on the preponderance of evidence showing the importance of sleep and the detrimental effect of lack of sleep, it's essential to make sleep a priority with a goal of 7-9 hours per night (47).

8. Remember that your taste buds will change over time. Much the way one's tolerance to alcohol changes with varying levels of alcohol intake, one's taste for sugar can change over time. To follow the alcohol analogy, a heavy drinker needs more alcohol to get drunk, while one who rarely drinks feel tipsy after one beer or glass of wine. The same is true with sugar. The soda drinker doesn't think fruit provides much sweetness, but after giving up soda, going back for a drink of soda, it tastes unpalatably sweet. As you start to limit your intake of sugar, you will start to have lower "tolerance" for sugar. Sweets you used to love will start to taste too sweet, and you will begin to enjoy the natural sweetness of fruit and foods like nuts that have a small amount of natural sweetness. Dark chocolate may even start to become enjoyable, when it may have seemed too bitter in the past.

9. Find your motivation. This is very important. Anytime you approach a new challenge, you need to be clear about your motivation. Do you want to lose weight? Have better energy or mood throughout the day? Are you concerned about your dental health? Do you want to better manage your diabetes or prevent it? The list could go on and on of why limiting sugar in your diet is important. Reread

Chapters 4 to 6 if you need motivation. Make sure you are clear what your individual motivation is. Write it down and return to that motivation when you feel your resolve slipping. Use motivational quotes and photos posted that help you remember why limiting sugar is so essential for you. You can do it, and it can become second nature to limit your sweets. It's just a matter of practice and hard work.

10. If you are struggling with motivation, make a pro/con list. I once worked with a client, who was struggling with weight loss. She was a recovering alcoholic who had been sober for many years, but struggled with cravings for sugar. We discussed setting limits on her sugar intake several times, but she would lose a few pounds, and then regain them because she would "lose control" around sugar. I asked her how she was feeling before her sugar binges, and she said it was usually when she was feeling lonely or sad. Then I asked her how overeating sweets was working as a coping mechanism for those feelings. Not so well, it turns out! We used this exercise from *The Pathway* by Lauren Mellein in which you essentially make a pro/con list for making the change and another pro/con list for not making the change. The pro is the "earned reward," and the con is the "essential pain (48)." You can use this with yourself, or if you are a healthcare provider, use it with your patients. It can help establish motivation and get through roadblocks. Let's use cutting out soda as an example.

Behavior change: Stop drinking soda

Earned Reward	Essential Pain
Lose weight	Not enjoying the flavor of soda
Less risk for diabetes and other chronic diseases	Feeling left out when others enjoy soda
Have more energy	Soda cravings
Feel better	Feeling lower energy at first
Look better	
Less sugar cravings	
Feel more in control of my life	

Alternative: Continue to drink soda

Earned Reward	Essential Pain
Continue to enjoy soda	Overweight
No extra effort to reduce soda intake	Higher risk for diabetes and other chronic diseases
	Continued reliance on sugar and caffeine for energy
	May continue to gain weight
	Feel unhappy about how I look
	Becoming harder to get around and do recreational activities

While these pros and cons may sound obvious, clearly writing out the pros and cons can be a very powerful motivator. My patient ended up coming back two months later after having lost 15 pounds and told me how powerful that exercise had been for her. She was able to limit her sugar intake and lose the weight. We often use eating, especially sweets, as a coping mechanism for stress, but afterward often feel worse than before. Finding alternative coping mechanisms like yoga, meditation, and productive distraction can be great ways to help you cope with these feelings instead of using sugar.

PART 3 KEY POINTS

1. Limit your added sugar intake to 10 grams/day or less. This is equivalent to 2.5 teaspoons of table sugar, 2 teaspoons of maple syrup, or 1 ½ teaspoons of honey daily.

2. Follow the 5-step process for weaning yourself off sugar:
　　1) Wean yourself off of all soda.
　　2) Eliminate all other sweetened beverages.
　　3) Scale back on desserts.
　　4) Limit non-dessert foods with added sugar.
　　5) Make sure you aren't overeating foods with naturally occurring sugars.

3. Follow my top 10 tips for kicking your sugar habit:
　　1) Never eat sweets on an empty stomach.
　　2) Eat more protein.
　　3) Brush your teeth after eating.
　　4) Practice productive distraction.
　　5) Avoid saboteurs.
　　6) Don't keep any sweets at home.
　　7) Get 7-9 hours of sleep per night.
　　8) Remember that your taste buds will change over time.
　　9) Find your motivation.
　　10) Make a pro/con list.

Part 4: How to Still Savor Some Sweetness

CHAPTER 10: WHYARTIFICIAL SWEETENERS ARE NOT THE ANSWER

Many people turn to artificial sweeteners as a substitute for sugar. It seems like a no-brainer – sweet taste without the calories and without the harmful effects of glucose or fructose. The problem is that most artificial sweeteners have other downsides. They only serve to exacerbate sugar cravings, and in the research don't necessarily help people lose weight. The current paradigm that assumes that diet sodas are okay because they don't contain any sugar is flawed, as artificial sweeteners may also have negative health effects.

In an article from researchers at the Harvard School of Public Health, the authors note that evidence indicates artificial sweeteners may increase sweet cravings and enhance appetite (49). In some striking research of more than 5,000 participants, at least daily consumption of diet soda was associated with a 37% increased risk of metabolic syndrome and 67% increased risk for diabetes (50)! Furthermore, in an analysis of data from the Nurse's Health Study, drinking 1 or more regular or diet sodas daily increased risk of having a stroke (51). One study that examined all artificial sweeteners noted an increased risk for pre-term labor with their use. Center for Science in the Public Interest (CSPI) recommends avoiding sucralose, aspartame, saccharin, and acesulfame K (52).

Sucralose: Generally known as Splenda, sucralose is manufactured by taking sugar and adding a chlorine molecule to it, which prevents absorption by the body. Given this chemical structure of sucralose, the idea that Splenda is "made from sugar, so it tastes like sugar" is quite misleading. A study done in mice suggests that sucralose may increase risk for leukemia (52). In addition, sucralose may affect the way your body responds to sugar. In a study of 17 subjects, the subjects either drank water or an equivalent volume of a beverage sweetened with sucralose (at the typical concentration of a 12-oz diet soda) and were then were given glucose 10 minutes later. The participants who consumed sucralose had a higher peak glucose response and a 20% higher insulin response compared to the water group. The results of this study demonstrate a potential mechanism by which artificial sweeteners could increase risk for diabetes and metabolic syndrome (53).

Aspartame: Aspartame is sold under the brands NutraSweet or Equal and is found in many diet sodas and "sugar-free" or "lite" foods. According to CSPI, three independent animal studies found that aspartame causes cancer in rodents. In my practice, some people with frequent headaches have found resolution when they quit aspartame. One mechanism by which some of the toxic effects of aspartame are thought to occur is that aspartame breaks down in the body to methanol, a toxic compound (52).

Saccharin: Saccharin is sold under the brand-name Sweet'N Low and has been associated with higher risk of bladder cancer in rodents as well as humans and is best avoided (52).

Acesulfame Potassium: Acesulfame potassium is found in chewing gum, baked goods, and diet sodas and is usually listed as acesulfame-K on the label. Acesulfame-K is frequently used along with sucralose. CSPI advises against using acesulfame-K due to inadequate safety testing and research suggesting acesulfame-K may increase cancer risk. CSPI also cites research noting that acesulfame K's breakdown products may be harmful to the thyroid based on data from animal studies (52).

Sugar Alcohols: This class of reduced calorie sweeteners, including maltitol, xylitol, erythritol, and mannitol are not well-absorbed by the body and thus have a lower calorie content than sugar. They are often a cause of diarrhea, and are thus not advised (52).

Truvia and PureVia: These stevia extracts are naturally derived, but I have chosen to discuss them along with artificial sweeteners since there is a high degree of processing in the creation of these calorie-free sweeteners. Truvia and PureVia are 95% or more rebaudioside A, a compound found naturally in the stevia leaf. In contrast whole leaf stevia contains both rebaudioside A and stevioside. These rebaudioside A extracts have been granted GRAS (generally recognized as safe) status by the FDA, but CSPI notes that safety testing was inadequate given concerns about the ability of rebaudioside A and derivatives to cause mutations (52). Truvia also contains erythritol and natural flavors. Erythritol is a sugar alcohol that is best avoided.

CHAPTER 11: THE BEST SWEETS AND SWEETENERS

The best options for sweets are those that are either naturally sweet or naturally nutrient-rich or both. Naturally sweet desserts include fruit smoothies, banana "ice cream," (see recipe section), and banana with natural peanut butter or almond butter. Dark chocolate, while it has added sugar, tends to be pretty low in sugar and is a rich source of minerals like iron and magnesium. In the accompanying chart, you can see that generally the higher the cocoa content, the lower the sugar content. Make sure to check the sugar content of chocolate, however, because as you can see Hershey's Special Dark has a whopping 21 grams of sugar despite being labeled a "dark" chocolate.

Sugar Content of Selected Dark Chocolate Brands

Dark Chocolate Brand	Sugar per 1.4 oz/40 gram serving (grams)
Lindt 90% cocoa	3
Lindt 85% cocoa	5
Green and Black's 85% cocoa	8
Green and Black's 70% cocoa	10
Endangered Species 72%	11
Hershey's Special Dark	21

Data from manufacturers' websites (current as of June 2013).

Many times people are advised to turn to high sugar sweets like jellybeans and gummy bears instead of high fat sweets like chocolate or ice cream. It's important to remember, and retrain your thinking that fat is not necessarily the enemy. Ten large jellybeans have 20 grams of sugar, no fat and no vitamins or minerals. Remember that the calorie and fat content aren't the only things that matter. The blood sugar spike provided by jellybeans leads to elevated insulin levels and increased fat storage, even though you're eating a non-fat food. That blood sugar spike and high sugar content of the jellybeans only serves to exacerbate sugar cravings and ignite a roller coaster of hunger, cravings, and crankiness.

Alternative Sweeteners to Refined Sugar

Using alternative sweeteners that have some nutrient and antioxidant value, though still providing sugar, is preferred over the use of white sugar, which completely lacks vitamins and minerals. Brown sugar, which many people think is more nutritious than white sugar, actually does not provide a significant amount of any vitamin or mineral. Brown sugar is brown due to the addition of molasses. Molasses is nutrient-rich, but the quantity added to make brown sugar isn't enough to give brown sugar any significant quantity of nutrients.

The summary below provides you with the type of sugar found in each sweetener along with potential health benefits or hazards, and nutrient content. The best choices are noted with an asterisk (*), but that is not encouragement to consume them in excess. Instead these are the best sweeteners to use *in small amounts.* You may have heard honey touted as a health food due to its ability to help with allergies. Eating a lot of honey still causes a blood sugar and insulin response, and you should remember that it contains sugar despite its benefits. For comparison, one teaspoon of white table sugar has 4 grams of total sugar in the form of sucrose.

*Honey: 6 grams total sugar per teaspoon
Honey is produced by those busy bees and contains about 50% fructose, which is still lower than 55% in HFCS and about the same fructose content as table sugar (15). Honey has anti-bacterial properties and is a source of antioxidants derived from the pollen collected by the bees. Darker honeys have higher antioxidant value. It's best to use raw or unprocessed honey for higher nutrient and antioxidant content (54).

*Maple Syrup: 4.5 grams total sugar per teaspoon
Not to be confused with Aunt Jemima "pancake syrup" that is made from HFCS and caramel coloring, real maple syrup is made by boiling the sap of maple or other trees into a concentrated and sweet syrup. People mostly associate maple syrup with pancakes and waffles, but maple syrup is a delicious sweetener for use in homemade ice cream, to sweeten some plain yogurt or in some lightly sweetened desserts. The sugar in maple syrup is predominantly sucrose. Maple syrup, especially grade B maple syrup, contains small amounts of calcium and zinc and a significant amount of riboflavin. One tablespoon of maple syrup provides about 20% of the daily requirement for riboflavin (15).

Agave Nectar: 5 grams total sugar per teaspoon
Agave nectar is the highest fructose sweetener, with at least 80% fructose (15). It has often been touted as a low glycemic index sweetener due to the low glucose content, but that high dose of fructose may increase triglycerides and fat synthesis by the liver and the storage of abdominal visceral fat (around the organs), which is associated with higher heart disease and diabetes risks. In my opinion, agave nectar is best avoided.

Brown rice syrup: 6 grams total sugar per teaspoon
Brown rice syrup is made by soaking, sprouting and cooking brown rice and enzymatically breaking down the

starch into maltose and other polymers of glucose (55). These sugars break down into 100% glucose. While inherently a good choice for a sweetener due to the lack of fructose, high arsenic levels have recently been found in rice, and the arsenic appears to concentrate in rice products like brown rice syrup, thus this sweetener is best limited. High intakes of arsenic may increase risk for skin, bladder, and lung cancer, according to the Environmental Working Group (56). It's important to note that arsenic compounds are divided into two groups – inorganic and organic. Inorganic arsenic is considered a known carcinogen, while organic arsenic is not considered as toxic as inorganic arsenic, but is noted to be a possible carcinogen. According to testing done by *Consumer Reports*, two tablespoons of brown rice syrup contains 4.6 to 5.9 micrograms of inorganic arsenic, while the federal limit for arsenic is 10 micrograms per 1 liter of drinking water, and New Jersey standards are less than 5 micrograms per liter of drinking water. *Consumer Reports* notes that arsenic comes from naturally occurring arsenic, use of arsenic-containing pesticides, and fertilizing with manure containing arsenic (57).

*Molasses: 5 grams total sugar per teaspoon

Molasses is the by-product of sugar cane refining and is a mixture of sucrose, glucose, and fructose. Molasses is perhaps the most nutrient-rich of all sweeteners. Molasses provides a significant amount of calcium, iron, magnesium, potassium, and vitamin B6. All of these nutrients are removed in the production of white sugar, which has no nutrients (15).

Whole Leaf Stevia: 0 grams total sugar per teaspoon

Stevia is a naturally derived sweetener from the yerba dulce plant that contains the chemicals stevioside and rebaudioside A, which give stevia its characteristic sweetness. Stevia is about 100 times sweeter than sugar. It has no calories or sugar at all. According to CSPI, stevia was rejected by the FDA as a food ingredient in the 1990s. Subsequently, rebaudioside A isolated from the stevia leaf (in Truvia and PureVia) has been given GRAS (Generally Recognized as Safe) status, which CSPI notes requires much less rigorous testing than approval as a food ingredient. Whole leaf stevia remains a dietary supplement as the FDA has still not approved it as food ingredient. Some of the concerns about whole leaf stevia are related to the fact that when high doses were fed to rats, their sperm production decreased. In addition, when high doses of whole leaf stevia were fed to pregnant hamsters, they had fewer and smaller offspring (52). Furthermore, stevia has the same problem that artificial sweeteners have in that it's so much sweeter than sugar and may exacerbate sugar cravings. My advice is to use whole leaf stevia sparingly, since the jury is still out on its safety.

*Dates: 16 grams total sugar per one medjool date

Dates are actually a fruit, but I think they deserve a place here, since they are so sweet and can help sweeten up desserts while still providing some nutritional value. The sugar in dates is a 50/50 mixture of fructose and glucose. You can think of one date as approximately equivalent in sugar content to one tablespoon (or 3 teaspoons) sugar. One date provides 5% of the daily requirement of vitamin B6 for adults and also contains small amounts of vitamin A, potassium, and calcium (15).

*Best choices

Other Sweeteners

There are multiple other less refined sweeteners that, like white sugar, are derived from sugar cane. These include turbinado, demerara, muscovado, and whole cane sugar. Whole cane sugar is often sold under the brand of "succanat (58)." These sweeteners have varying degrees of refining with whole cane sugar and muscovado having the highest molasses content, meaning higher nutrient content (59). Coconut sugar is another sweetener that is becoming more widely available, and is made from the nectar of the coconut flower blossom. Date sugar is another option and is made from ground and dehydrated dates, so date sugar will contain similar vitamins and minerals to fresh dates. Unfortunately, there is little to no data on the nutrient content or glycemic index or load of the majority of these sweeteners, but those for which there is data are listed here.

Glycemic Index and Glycemic Load of Sweeteners

Sweetener	Glycemic Index	Serving size	Glycemic Load
White sugar	60	1 tablespoon	6
Honey	58	1 tablespoon	3
Maple syrup	54	1 tablespoon	2
Dates	47	1 date	8
Agave nectar	11	1 tablespoon	1

Data from glycemicindex.com (16).

What to Look For in a Sweetener
1. Naturally derived.
2. 50% or less of the sugar is fructose.
3. Contains nutrients and/or antioxidants.
4. Minimally processed.
5. Not contaminated with pesticides/toxins.
6. No potential health risks.

When we use these six criteria in evaluating a sweetener, number one eliminates the artificial sweeteners discussed previously since they are chemically synthesized. High fructose intake can increase fat synthesis and may lead to fatty liver and more difficulty achieving weight loss. If that's your goal it's best to steer clear of higher fructose sweeteners like agave nectar. The most nutrient-rich sweetener is molasses, which is a great choice. Honey and maple syrup also contain some nutrients and antioxidants, as do dates. Many derivatives of sugar cane, even if they are natural, are quite refined and stripped of nutrients. When all is said and done, honey, maple syrup, molasses, and dates are the best options. Fruit is another good option, of course, that has varying content of total sugars, sucrose, fructose, and glucose.

CHAPTER 12: SWEET FREEDOM

Throughout the course of this book, I've covered the basic information about sugar in order to educate you about how sugar breaks down and affects your body. I hope I have convinced you that added sugar in your diet has some very real health risks. These negative health effects seem increasingly to be related to fructose, but are related to the actions of glucose as well.

People will often say "everything in moderation" when referring to eating patterns. This really isn't helpful, since it begs the question what is a "moderate" amount of sugar? As we now know, the average daily sugar consumption in the US is really quite high. Health agencies and the US government have been hesitant to make very specific recommendations on sugar consumption. When they do make recommendations, they simply, in my opinion, do not go far enough. I recommend daily maximum of 10 grams of added sugar. While a lofty goal, it is a worthy goal, as your long-term health and vitality may depend on it.

Whether your goal is to lose weight, decrease belly fat, improve your blood sugar regulation, or have fewer mood swings or more consistent energy levels, I challenge you to cut the sugar out of your diet and see what happens. I suspect that, over time, you will feel better than you have ever felt and will drop the excess weight and cut your risk of disease.

Following a step-wise approach to cutting your sugar intake provides a systematic way to approach behavior change and increases the likelihood of success. Be sure to set specific and measurable goals. Let's use the example of someone with a 12-oz. daily soda habit. In the first week you could cut back to three 12-oz. sodas for the week. If you achieve that goal, you cut it down further in subsequent weeks. Make sure to celebrate your successes, and try to find the root of your cravings and slip-ups. For more information and helpful resources to help you on your journey, check out sugarbreaker.com.

Over time, the goal is to wean yourself to very little or no added sugar on most days. On those occasions when you do have sweets, choose small amounts of natural sweeteners, or savor a square of dark chocolate or a small bowl of real ice cream. On most days, fruit should be your source of sweetness. When you are used to eating sweets frequently, fruit just doesn't taste as sweet. Decreasing your sugar intake has many rewards, including improved health and decreased disease risk. A more immediate benefit is a newfound ability to derive pleasure from the delicate sweetness of strawberries or a juicy summer peach.

PART 4 KEY POINTS

1. Avoid all artificial sweeteners including sucralose (Splenda), aspartame, saccharin, acesulfame-K, and sugar alcohols. Each of these sweeteners has health risks including possible increased cancer risk, digestive and thyroid problems, and dysfunctional blood sugar regulation.

2. Limit agave nectar due to its high fructose content. Limit brown rice syrup due to concerns about arsenic contamination.

3. The best natural substitutes for white table sugar are honey, maple syrup, molasses, and dates.

No Sugar and Very Low Sugar Recipes

DESERTS

Vanilla Coconut Macaroons
These macaroons are a delectable treat and can be made in under 5 minutes!

1/8 cup almond flour
1/8 cup shredded coconut
1 teaspoon maple syrup
¼ teaspoon vanilla

Mix all ingredients together in a small bowl until well moistened. Form into balls and enjoy! Macaroons will hold together better after refrigeration.

Makes 3 servings
Sugar Content per serving: 1.5 grams total sugar as sucrose, 1.5 grams added sugar

Cashew Cream
This delicious low-sugar and dairy-free "cream" makes fruit taste like a delectable treat. Use this cashew cream to make dairy-free strawberry ice cream.
Adapted from Nut Cream in *Feeding the Whole Family* (55).

½ cup raw unsalted cashews
1 tablespoon maple syrup
1 teaspoon vanilla
1 ½ teaspoons water

Pulse cashews in food processor into a fine meal. Add maple syrup and vanilla and process further. Slowly add water and process further until you have a thick cream.

Makes 4 servings
Sugar Content per serving: 3.4 grams total sugar as sucrose, 3.4 grams added sugar

Dairy-free Strawberry Ice Cream
This dairy-free and very low sugar ice cream will amaze you with the gentle sweetness of banana and cashew cream.

1 banana
½ cup raw unsalted cashews
1 tablespoon maple syrup
1 teaspoon vanilla
1 ½ teaspoons water
1 cup frozen strawberries
Cashew cream (see recipe above)

Peel and slice banana into ½ inch thick slices, and arrange on a plate, and place in the freezer for 1-2 hours. Before banana slices are ready to come out of the freezer, pulse cashews in food processor into a fine meal. Add maple syrup, vanilla, and water and process further until you have a thick cashew cream. Remove cashew cream from food processor and clean food processor. Add frozen banana slices and strawberries and puree until well blended. Add cashew cream and process until smooth and creamy. Store in the freezer. Enjoy!

Makes about 3 half-cup servings
Sugar Content per serving: 10.4 grams total sugar, 6.5 grams sucrose, 1.9 grams fructose, 2 grams glucose, 4.5 grams added sugar

Chocolate Banana Ice Cream
Adapted from the Kitchn's Magic One Ingredient Ice Cream (60). This deliciously creamy and chocolaty ice cream is just as good as the real thing with no added sugar. The sugar content is the naturally occurring sugar in the bananas.

2 bananas
¼ cup cocoa powder
2 tablespoons heavy cream
1 teaspoon vanilla

Peel and slice bananas into ½ inch thick slices, and arrange on a plate and place in the freezer for 1-2 hours. Blend bananas in the food processor until smooth and creamy. Add cocoa powder, cream, and vanilla and blend thoroughly. Store in the freezer.

Makes about 3 half-cup servings
Sugar Content per serving: 9.6g total sugar, 1 gram sucrose, 3.8 grams fructose, 3.9 grams glucose, 0 grams added sugar

Superfood Bars
Enjoy these delicious nutrient-dense bars for breakfast on-the-go, an afternoon energy boost, or a satisfying healthy dessert.

8 oz. (half a 16-oz. jar) natural peanut butter
½ cup honey
½ cup chia seeds
1/8 cup organic spirulina
½ cup cocoa powder
½ cup shredded unsweetened coconut
Combine peanut butter and honey in a medium-sized bowl. Mix in remaining ingredients until evenly distributed. Press into a standard-sized loaf pan. Refrigerate overnight. Cut into 24 equal sized bars.

Makes 24 servings
Sugar Content per serving: 6 grams total sugar, 0.5 grams sucrose, 2.9 grams fructose, 2.6 grams glucose, 5.7 grams added sugar

BEVERAGES

Cucumber Water
This refreshing beverage is a great way to stay hydrated with the gentle flavor of cucumber.

4 cups filtered water
6+ slices cucumber

Add cucumber to a pitcher of water and allow to infuse overnight in the refrigerator. You can choose to leave the cucumber slices in the water or remove them.

Makes 4 servings
Sugar Content per serving: 0 grams total sugar

Cold Brewed Green Tea with Pomegranate Juice
This antioxidant-rich drink derives its delicate sweetness from a splash of pomegranate juice

1-2 teaspoons of loose green tea or 1-2 teabags
4 cups filtered water
½ cup pomegranate juice

Infuse green tea bags or loose tea in an infuser in water overnight in the refrigerator. Remove tea and add pomegranate juice in the morning.

Makes 4 servings
Sugar Content per serving: 4 grams total sugar, 2 grams fructose, 2 grams glucose, 0 grams added sugar

Green Juice
This vegetable juice is full of detoxifying chlorophyll as well as antioxidants like beta-carotene.

4 organic medium carrots
4 organic celery stalks
3 leaves organic kale
3 mint sprigs

Wash all vegetables thoroughly and cut off ends of carrots, celery. Juice all vegetables in juicer.

Makes 1 serving
Sugar content per serving: 14.5 grams total sugar, 8.8 grams sucrose, 2.2 grams fructose, 2.2 grams glucose, 0 grams added sugar

REFERENCES

1. WHO Definition of Health. World Health Organization website. Available at:
http://www.who.int/about/definition/en/print.html. Accessed July 2013.
2. US Consumption of Caloric Sweeteners. USDA Economic Research Service. Available at:
http://www.ers.usda.gov/data-products/sugar-and-sweeteners-yearbook-tables.aspx#25512. Accessed July 2013.
3. Dietary Guidelines for Americans 2010. US Dept. of Health and Human Services. Available at:
http://www.health.gov/dietaryguidelines/dga2010/DietaryGuidelines2010.pdf. Accessed July 2013.
4. Saad L. To Lose Weight, Americans Rely More on Dieting Than Exercise. Gallup Wellness. 2011. Available at
http://www.gallup.com/poll/150986/lose-weight-americans-rely-dieting-exercise.aspx. Accessed July 2012.
5. Bittman M. It's the Sugar Folks. New York Times Opinionator. 2013. Available at
http://opinionator.blogs.nytimes.com/2013/02/27/its-the-sugar-folks/. Accessed July 2013.
6. Nestle M. NYC Health Department: One New Yorker Dies of Diabetes Every 90 minutes. Food Politics Blog. 2013. Available at
http://www.foodpolitics.com/2013/06/nyc-health-department-one-new-yorker-dies-of-diabetes-every-90-minutes/. Accessed July 2013.
7. Gropper SS, Smith JL, Groff JL. *Advanced Nutrition and Human Metabolism.* 4th ed. Belmont, CA: Thomson Wadsworth; 2005.
8. Herbicides. Environmental Protection Agency. Available at http://www.epa.gov/caddis/ssr_herb_int.html. Accessed July 2013.
9. Pollan M. The Omnivore's Dilemma: A Natural History of Four Meals. New York: Penguin Group; 2006.

10. Maersk M, Belza A, Stødkilde-Jørgensen H et al. Sucrose-sweetened beverages increase fat storage in the liver, muscle and visceral fat depot: a 6-mo randomized intervention study. *Am J Clin Nutr.*2012;95(2):283-289.

11. Richelsen B. Sugar-sweetened beverages and cardio-metabolic disease risks. *Curr Opin Clin Nutr Metab Care.* 2013;16(4):478-484.

12. Aeberli I, Hochuli M, Gerber PA et al. Moderate amounts of fructose consumption impair insulin sensitivity in healthy young men. *Diabetes Care.* 2013;36:150-156.

13. Bravo S, Lowndes J, Sinnett S, Yu Z, Rippe J. Consumption of sucrose and high-fructose corn syrup does not increase liver fat or ectopic fat accumulation in muscles. *Appl Physiol Nutr Metab.* 2013;38:681-688.

14. Ha V, Jayalath VH, Cozma AI, Mirrahimi A, de Souza RJ, Sievenpiper JL. Fructose-containing sugars, blood Pressure, and cardiometabolic risk: a critical review. *Curr Hypertens Rep.* June 22, 2013. Epub ahead of print.

15. USDA National Nutrient Database for Standard Reference, Release 25. US Department of Agriculture, Agricultural Research Service. 2012. Available at http://www.ars.usda.gov/ba/bhnrc/ndl. Accessed June-July 2013.

16. Glycemic Index Database: University of Sydney. Available at http://glycemicindex.com. Accessed July 2013.

17. Foster-Powell K, Holt SH, Brand-Miller JC. International table of glycemic index and load values: 2002. *Am J Clin Nutr.* 2002;76(10):5-56.

18. Lustig RH, Schmidt LA, Brindis CD. Public health: The toxic truth about sugar. *Nature.* 2012;482(7383):27-29.

19. Stanhope KL, Schwarz JM, Havel PJ. Adverse metabolic effects of dietary fructose: results from the recent epidemiological, clinical, and mechanistic studies. *Curr Opin Lipidol.* 2013;24(3):198-206.

20. Diagnosing Diabetes and Learning About Prediabetes. American Diabetes Association. Available at:

http://www.diabetes.org/diabetes-basics/diagnosis/.
Accessed July 2013.

21. Mahan K, Escott-Stump S. *Krause's Food, Nutrition, &*
Diet Therapy. 11th ed. Philadelphia, PA: Elsevier; 2004.

22. Diabetes Myths. American Diabetes Association.
Available at: http://www.diabetes.org/diabetes-
basics/diabetes-myths/?loc=DropDownDB-myths.
Accessed July 2013.

23. Malik VS, Popkin BM, Bray GA, Deprés JP, Willett WC,
Hu FB. Sugar-sweetened beverages and risk of metabolic
syndrome and type 2 diabetes: a meta-analysis. *Diabetes Care.*
2010;33(11):2477-2483.

24. Basu S, Yoffe P, Hills N, Lustig RN. The relationship of
sugar to population-level diabetes prevalence: an
econometric analysis of repeated cross-sectional data. *PLoS*
One. 2013;8(2):e357873. Epub ahead of print.

25. Living with Diabetes: Heart Disease. American Diabetes
Association. Available at http://www.diabetes.org/living-
with-diabetes/complications/heart-disease/. Accessed July
2013.

26. Lockhart PB, Bolger AF, Papapanou PN et al.
Periodontal disease and atherosclerotic vascular disease: dose
the evidence supports a independent association?: A
scientific statement from the American Heart Association.
Circulation. 2012;125(20):2520-2544.

27. Spreadbury I. Comparison with ancestral diets suggests
dense acellular carbohydrates promote an inflammatory
microbiota, and may be the primary dietary cause of leptin
resistance and obesity. *Diabetes Metab Syndr Obes.* 2012;5:175-
189.

28. Metabolic Syndrome: Tests and diagnosis. Mayo Clinic.
Available at
http://www.mayoclinic.com/health/metabolic%20syndrom
e/DS00522/DSECTION=tests-and-diagnosis. Accessed
July 2013.

29. Cancer Facts and Figures. American Cancer Society.
Available at

http://www.cancer.org/acs/groups/content/@epidemiolog ysurveilance/documents/document/acspc-036845.pdf. Accessed July 2013.

30. Stay Healthy. American Cancer Society. Available at: http://www.cancer.org/healthy/index. Accessed July 2013.

31. Body Composition, Growth, and Development: Food, Nutrition, Physical Activity and the Prevention of Cancer: World Cancer Research Fund and American Institute for Cancer Research. Available at http://www.dietandcancerreport.org/cancer_resource_cente r/downloads/chapters/chapter_06.pdf. Accessed July 2013.

32. Experts Explore Emerging Evidence Linking Diabetes and Cancer. American Diabetes Association. Available at http://www.diabetes.org/for-media/2010/experts-explore-emerging-evidence-linking-diabetes-and-cancer.html. Accessed July 2013.

33. Gunter MJ, Hoover DR, Yu H et al. Insulin, insulin-like growth factor-I, and risk of breast cancer in postmenopausal women. *J Natl Cancer Inst.* 2009;101:48-60.

34. Kabat GC, Kim M, Caan BJ. Repeated measures of serum glucose and insulin in relation to postmenopausal breast cancer. *Int J Cancer.* 2009;125(11):2704-2710.

35. Shikany JM, Redden DT, Neuhouser ML et al. Dietary glycemic load, glycemic index, and carbohydrate and risk of breast cancer in the Women's Health Initiative. *Nutr Cancer.* 2011;63(6):899-907.

36. King MG, Chandran U, Olson SH et al. Consumption of sugary foods and drinks and risk of endometrial cancer. *Cancer Causes Control.*2013;24(7):1427-1436.

37. Drake I, Sonestedt E, Gullberg B et al. Dietary intake of carbohydrates in relation to prostate cancer risk: a prospective study in the Mälmo Diet and Cancer cohort. *Am J Clin Nutr.* 2012;96(6):1409-1418.

38. Richman EL, Kenfield SA, Chavarro JE et al. Fat intake after diagnosis and risk of lethal prostate cancer and all-cause mortality. *JAMA Intern Med.* Jun 10, 2013. Epub ahead of print.

39. Caso J, Masko EM, Ii JA et al. The effect of carbohydrate restriction on prostate cancer tumor growth in a castrate mouse xenograft model. *Prostate*. 2013;73(5):449-454.
40. Theodoratou E, Farrington SM, Tenesa A et al. Associations between dietary and lifestyle factors and colorectal cancer in the Scottish population. *Eur J Cancer Prev*. Jun 28, 2013. Epub ahead of print.
41. Meyerhardt JA, Sato K, Niedzwiecki D et al. Dietary glycemic load and cancer recurrence and survival in patients with stage III colon cancer: Findings from CALGB 89803. *J Natl Cancer Inst*. 2012;104(22)1702-1711.
42. What are Empty Calories: USDA Choose MyPlate.gov. Available at http://www.choosemyplate.gov/weight-management-calories/calories/empty-calories.html. Accessed July 2013.
43. Summary of the ACS Guidelines on Nutrition and Physical Activity. American Cancer Society. 2012. Available at http://www.cancer.org/healthy/eathealthygetactive/acsguidelinesonnutritionphysicalactivityforcancerprevention/acs-guidelines-on-nutrition-and-physical-activity-for-cancer-prevention-summary. Accessed July 2013.
44. Healthy Eating. American Diabetes Association. Available at http://www.diabetes.org/diabetes-basics/prevention/checkup-america/healthy-eating.html. Accessed July 2013.
45. Frequently Asked Questions About Sugar: American Heart Association. Available at http://www.heart.org/HEARTORG/GettingHealthy/NutritionCenter/HealthyDietGoals/Frequently-Asked-Questions-About-Sugar_UCM_306725_Article.jsp. Accessed July 18, 2013.
46. Markwald RR, Melanson EL, Smith MR et al. Impact of insufficient sleep on total daily energy expenditure, food intake, and weight gain. *Proc Natl Acad Sci USA*. 2013;110(14):5695-5700.

47. Broussard JL, Ehrmann DA, Van Cauter E, Tasali E, Brady MJ. Impaired insulin signaling in human adipocytes after experimental sleep restriction: A randomized, crossover study. *Ann of Intern Med.* 2012;157(8):549-557.
48. Mellin L. The Pathway: *Follow the Road to Health and Happiness.* New York: Regan Books; 2003.
49. Malik VS, Hu FB. Sweeteners and risk of obesity and type 2 diabetes: the role of sugar-sweetened beverages. *Curr Diab Rep.* 2012;12:195-203.
50. Nettleton JA, Lutsey PL, Wang Y, Lima JA, Michose ED, Jacobs DR. Diet soda intake and risk of incident metabolic syndrome and type 2 diabetes in the multi-ethnic study of atherosclerosis (MESA). *Diabetes Care.* 2009;32(4):688-694.
51. Bernstein AM, de Konig L, Flint AJ, Rexrode KM, Willet WC. Soda consumption and the risk of stroke in men and women. *Am J Clin Nutr.* 2012;95:1190-1199.
52. Chemical Cuisine: Learn about Food Additives. Center for Science in the Public Interest. Available at http://www.cspinet.org/reports/chemcuisine.htm#artificial sweeteners. Accessed July 2013.
53. Pepino MY, Tiemann CD, Patterson BW, Wice BM, Klein S. Sucralose affects glycemic and hormonal responses to an oral glucose load. *Diabetes Care.* April 30, 2013. Epub ahead of print
54. Honey. Natural Medicine Comprehensive Database. Available at http://naturaldatabase.therapeuticresearch.com/nd/Search.aspx?cs=ONDPG&s=ND&pt=9&Product=honey&btnSearch.x=0&btnSearch.y=0. Accessed June 25, 2013.
55. Lair C. *Feeding the Whole Family: Whole Foods Recipes for Babies, Young Children and Their Parents.* Rev ed. Seattle, WA: Moon Smile Press; 1997.
56. Lunder S, Undurraga D. Getting Arsenic Out Of Your (And Your Kids' Diet). Environmental Working Group. 2012. Available at

http://www.ewg.org/enviroblog/2012/09/getting-arsenic-out-your-and-your-kids-diet. Accessed July 2013.
57. Arsenic in Your Food. 2012. Consumer Reports. Available at
http://www.consumerreports.org/cro/magazine/2012/11/arsenic-in-your-food/index.htm. Accessed August 2013.
58. Christensen E. What's the Difference? Muscovado, Demerara, & Turbinado. 2011. The Kitchn. Available at http://www.thekitchn.com/whats-the-difference-muscovado-145157. Accessed July 2013.
59. Velden D. Ingredient Spotlight: Dark Brown Muscovado Brown Sugar. The Kitchn. 2010. Available at http://www.thekitchn.com/ingredient-spotlight-dark-brow-115399. Accessed July 2013.
60. How to Make Creamy Ice Cream with Just One Ingredient. The Kitchn. 2011. Available at http://www.thekitchn.com/how-to-make-creamy-ice-cream-w-93414. Accessed July 2013.

ABOUT THE AUTHOR

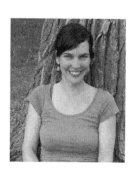

Margaret Wertheim is a Nutritionist and Registered Dietitian (RD) who specializes in helping people break the sugar habit. Margaret holds a BS in Biochemistry from the University of Wisconsin-Madison and an MS in Nutrition from Bastyr University in Seattle. Margaret has written or been quoted in numerous articles on nutrition, such as in Kiwi magazine, Today's Dietitian, Pregnancy and Newborn, and MindBodyGreen. Margaret's recipes, articles on sugar, natural sweeteners, and inflammation have been shared thousands of times. When she's not writing or working with clients, you can find her doing yoga, gardening, riding her bike, or experimenting in the kitchen. Check out her website at MargaretWertheimRD.com.

Made in the USA
Middletown, DE
12 April 2016